HOLISTIC MEDICAL TREATMENT OPTIONS FOR CHRONIC BLADDER AND INTERSTITIAL CYSTITIS PAIN

Copyright 2016 - All rights reserved.

This document is geared towards providing exact and reliable information in regards to the topic and issue covered. The publication is sold with the idea that the publisher is not required to render accounting, officially permitted, or otherwise, qualified services. If advice is necessary, legal or professional, a practiced individual in the profession should be ordered.

From a Declaration of Principles which was accepted and approved equally by a Committee of the American Bar Association and a Committee of Publishers and Associations.

In no way is it legal to reproduce, duplicate, or transmit any part of this document in either electronic means or in printed format. Recording of this publication is strictly prohibited and any storage of this document is not allowed unless with written permission from the publisher. All rights reserved.

The information provided herein is stated to be truthful and consistent, in that any liability, in terms of inattention or otherwise, by any usage or abuse of any policies, processes, or directions contained within is the solitary and utter responsibility of the recipient reader. Under no circumstances will any legal responsibility or blame be held against the publisher for any reparation, damages, or monetary loss due to the information herein, either directly or indirectly.

Respective authors own all copyrights not held by the publisher.

The information herein is offered for informational purposes solely, and is universal as so. The presentation of the information is without contract or any type of guarantee assurance.

The trademarks that are used are without any consent, and the publication of the trademark is without permission or backing by the trademark owner. All trademarks and brands within this book are for clarifying purposes only and are the owned by the owners themselves, not affiliated with this document.

CONTENTS

Introduction vii
   Is This book for me? ix
Chapter 1: What Is Interstitial Cystitis (IC)? 1
Chapter 2: What can cause IC? 7
   Autoimmune 8
   Hereditary 8
   Hormones 9
   Neurogenic 11
   Infectious 12
Symptoms of IC 13
   Painful Urination and/or Bladder Pain 13
   Sexual difficulties 15
   Frequent need to urinate 15
   Other bladder related symptoms 15
   Non-bladder related symptoms 16
Chapter 3: What are my options? 18
   DIET! DIET! DIET! 18
   Modify your diet 19
   Understand your triggers 20
   Elimination diet 20
   Alkalize 31
   ALKALIZING FOODS 34
   ACIDIFYING FOODS 37
Chapter 4: Not getting better with ic diet, why??? 39

Chapter 5: Ease the pain 44
    Alkalize on the spot 44
  Drink this 44
  Supplements 45
  Don't fall for diet scams 48
  Should I pee often or hold it in? 48
  Physical Therapy 50
  Smoking/Tobacco 50
  Exercise 51
  Meditate 52
  Use Heat/bath in lavender or Epsom salt 52
  Acupuncture 53
  NAET 53

Chapter 6: Medical Route 55
  What's wrong with IC patients medically speaking? 55
  Potassium sensitivity test 55
  Doctor's Visit 57
  Urine test 57
  Antibiotics 58
  MRI 58
  Cystoscopy 59
  Biopsy 60
  Oral medications 60
  Over the counter 60
  Antihistamines: 60
  Antidepressants 61
  ELmiron 62
  Nerve stimulation techniques 64
  Transcutaneous electrical nerve stimulation (TENS). 64
  Sacral nerve stimulation 65

Bladder distention 65
Bladder Drug Instillation (Bladder Wash) 66
DMSO 68
New Emerging Studies 68
Resiniferatoxin 69
Hyaluronic Acid 69
Hydrodistention/Hyaluronic Acid 70
Intravesical bacillus Calmette-Guérin 71
Intravesical liposomes 71
Hyperbaric Oxygen 72
Corticosteroids Silver nitrate 72
Sodium oxychlorosene 72
Immunosuppressives Heparin 73
Surgery 73
Fulguration 74
Resection 74
Bladder augmentation 74

Conclusion 75
STICK TO IT AND GIVE IT TIME!!! 75

INTRODUCTION

I want to thank you and congratulate you for downloading this book. You've now taken the first step in taking control of this disease and taking back your life.

I have been struggling with this ailment for over twenty years! I have tried many things, most of which have not worked. Some treatments took me years to realize that they were futile, i.e. cranberry juice and vitamin C could be flaring up my Interstitial Cystitis (IC) problems instead of healing them. I tried hundreds of trial and error approaches to relieve symptoms. I have researched online, read books, joined forums and joined support groups, having learned many things during my journey. I've designed this book to have multi-faceted approach in dealing with IC, having realized that not all things work for everyone as all of our bodies are different. However, I've focused in on treatments that have been known to be the most effective in my opinion, including both traditional medical and non-traditional treatments.

I recommend you consider both routes, alternative/holistic approach and more conventional/medical approach…so that you can better determine what works best for you. Keep in mind, this is a journey that will take some time, it is not a quick solution so please, don't give up. However I will guide you through easy pain management steps to help you along the way.

I know it's hard to believe, but you are not alone. When I tried treatments that did not work, or when I heard from my physician yet again that taking antibiotics and cranberry extract juice would "make it go away" and after decades of antibiotics after antibiotics, doing me more harm than good (ruining my intestinal flora), I became frustrated and depressed. I finally made the decision to take control of my life and this disease, once and for all.

It's important to note, I am not a medical professional of any kind. I am simply a person that has suffered with this disease for years on end and have decided to put all of the knowledge I have accumulated over the years in this book with the hopes of helping others suffering as I have for so many years. In this book you'll find medical information, alternative approaches, proper diet strategies and simple tricks on how to ease Interstitial Cystitis pain for the short-term and methods to help heal you of this disease. My only intention here is to help others like me deal with this disease.

IS THIS BOOK FOR ME?

If you've been dealing with pain during urination, bladder pain, pelvic pain without relief in sight, having tried several methods but have not found a short or long term cure, this book is for you. A range of treatment options for Interstitial Cystitis exist, from changing diet, to exercising, alternative treatments to traditional medical options such as medication, procedures and surgeries. Each alternative and medical treatment comes with its own set of benefits and drawbacks. The strategies outlined in this book approach IC with alternative as well as medical treatments. The strategies in this book are aimed to make you feel better, and to give you an array of options to help get you on the road to recovery.

CHAPTER 1

WHAT IS INTERSTITIAL CYSTITIS (IC)?

Interstitial Cystitis affects more than a million people in the United States, mostly women. However it is known to affect men as well.

IC symptoms can be similar to those of a bladder infection, but the difference is that IC patients will have sterile urine. Thus far, research points to a damaged bladder lining as the biggest culprit behind IC.

The bladder is a hollow balloon-like organ that collects urine from the kidneys and holds it until it can be expelled. The walls of the bladder consist mainly of muscle that relaxes as the bladder fills and contracts to empty it. The inside walls are covered with a lining of cells that protect the muscle from contact with urine. The bladder expands until it's full and then signals your brain that it's time to urinate, communicating through the pelvic nerves. This creates the urge to urinate for most people. With Interstitial Cystitis, these signals get mixed up — you feel the need to urinate more often and with smaller volumes of urine than most people.

Inflammation is a protective reaction of the body tissue to irritation, injury, or infection. Inflammation of the bladder is called cystitis. When the inflammation is caused by bacterial infection, it is referred to as bacterial cystitis or just cystitis. Interstitial Cystitis(IC) is a condition that causes pain and inflammation in the bladder when no infection is found. (Other causes of noninfectious inflammation of the bladder are also possible.)

This type of inflammation of the bladder causes urinary frequency (frequent need to urinate), urgency (urgent need to urinate), pelvic pain, painful urination, incontinence, and nocturia (frequent need to urinate at night).

Long-term inflammation of the bladder in people with IC can lead to scarring and stiffening of the bladder wall, which causes a decrease in the bladder capacity. Pinpoint areas of bleeding, called glomerulations, may occur in the lining of the bladder wall. IC is believed to be a syndrome initially presenting with mild symptoms and progressing to severe urgency and pelvic pain.

IC is a condition that consists of recurring pelvic pain, pressure, or discomfort in the bladder and pelvic region, often associated with urinary pain, frequency and urgency.

IC also goes by many other names, including painful bladder syndrome, bladder pain syndrome, hypersensitive syndrome, and pelvic floor dysfunction. Interstitial Cystitis is basically a chronic inflammation of the bladder that causes chronic pain and discomfort.

According to the IC Association, 90% of IC patients are said to have nonulcerative IC, which is marked by pinpoint hemorrhages in the bladder wall. The other 10% have ulcerative IC, which is named for the Hunner's ulcers, or red, bleeding patches found on the bladder wall.

According to the National Institutes of Health (NIH), IC is more common in women. It is believed that many patients have early forms of IC with a delayed diagnosis. The average age of onset of IC is 40 years.

Interstitial Cystitis can result in a number of complications, including:

Reduced bladder capacity

Interstitial Cystitis can lead to a stiffening of the wall of your bladder and reduced bladder capacity, meaning your bladder holds less urine.

Lower quality of life

Frequent urination and pain may interfere with social activities, work and other activities of daily life.

Sexual intimacy problems

Frequent urination and pain may strain your personal relationships, and sexual intimacy is commonly affected.

Emotional troubles

The chronic pain and interrupted sleep associated with Interstitial Cystitis may cause emotional stress and can lead to depression.

Interstitial Cystitis can be intolerable. It could hamper your life completely from engaging in normal day to day activity. You will find yourself planning trips around bathrooms, sex life can be non-existent, most of the time you just live with it. It's hard to diagnose, often it takes a very long time to properly have it diagnosed. It is because there are many more likely causes to your bladder pain than IC, making it more difficult for a doctor to diagnose. IC patients are at first, more commonly treated for a Urinary Tract Infection (UTI), Vaginitis, STD's: Chlamydia, Herpes, Kidney Stones, Endometriosis, Bladder Cancer, Diabetes, Prostatitis, etc.

These disorders have different root causes and need different types of treatments. Many women with IC see their healthcare practitioners thinking they have a UTI and are told their urine is "clean," meaning in the urine culture obtained, no abnormalities were found when it was evaluated in the lab. If there is no detected "problem," it frequently means that there simply is no easy solution. Because the symptoms of IC are similar to those of other disorders of the urinary system, the first step is to rule out other diseases before considering a diagnosis of IC. As more medical professionals learn to identify the IC conditions, they are better able to help manage as well as overcome this disorder. The Interstitial Cystitis Association and the Interstitial Cystitis Network are wonderful organizations that are promoting more awareness of the varied causes and symptoms so more people can get relief.

Once you have ruled out other diseases and have confirmed your IC diagnoses you can begin your road to recovery!

CHAPTER 2

WHAT CAN CAUSE IC?

Although many theories have been put forward, the cause of IC is unknown. Anyone can develop Interstitial Cystitis at any age. IC is most common, though, in women. It generally develops in middle age, and many people with IC also have other pain-related conditions, such as irritable bowel syndrome or fibromyalgia.

Other than being female, there are no known factors that increase the risk for Interstitial Cystitis. Consequently, there is no known way to prevent it or to prevent the symptoms from recurring after it goes into remission.In fact, because IC varies from person to person, scientists believe there may be multiple causes.

What is clearly understood though is that inflammation is at play, with possible immune dysfunction, specifically allergies and sensitivities, having a central role.

Here are a few possibilities:

AUTOIMMUNE

An autoimmune response is a physical response in which cells and antibodies of a person's body are directed against that person's own tissues. An autoimmune response to a bladder infection destroys the lining of the bladder wall. An unexplained association of IC has been found to exist with other autoimmune diseases such as inflammatory bowel disease, systemic lupus erythematosus, scleroderma, Sjogren syndrome, fibromyalgia, and atopic allergy. IC has a very high association with disorders of the bowel such as inflammatory bowel disease.

HEREDITARY

Studies of mothers, daughters, and twins who have IC suggest a hereditary risk factor. However, no gene has yet been implicated as a cause of IC.

Mast cell abnormalities: An overproduction of histamine and other potentially harmful chemicals by mast cells, a special type of cell that normally protects the body from allergic reactions. In some people with IC, special white blood cells called mast cells (associated with inflammation) are found in the bladder lining. Mast cells release histamine and other chemicals that cause inflammation of the bladder.

Studies have shown that some of the contents found typically in our urine (like potassium, for example) can infiltrate the bladder lining in IC patients, leading to mast cell activation and the release of histamine — which can then result in further damage to the bladder lining and amplified inflammation. More than 70% of women with IC have highly activated mast cells. Again this is an example of the inflammatory system being on high alert. A reduction in estrogen levels can activate our mast cells. Estrogen is an anti-inflammatory agent.

HORMONES

Balance your hormones. Some notice their first symptoms are during the premenopausal time frame. This could be due to estrogen levels.

Estrogen plays a significant role in inflammation, and during times of great hormonal imbalances your body could be more susceptible to inflammation that can lead to Interstitial Cystitis. Consider a natural approach to hormonal balance in your system, such as a soy supplement. When evaluating bladder mast cells researchers at Tufts (this needs to be sourced. Any research reference should be sourced either at the bottom or end of the document) who examined the mast cells under an electron microscope also noticed a large number of estrogen receptors in cells from women with IC. The net result in these women is similar to hormones that are imbalanced. They described this as similar to a progesterone deficient state which lead to increased mast cell secretion of histamine. This is the body's immune response to an offender.

In looking at the bladder's anatomy, the bladder lining and the muscle that essentially governs urination, the detrusor, are greatly affected by inflammation, mast cell activity, and estrogen. If we have ongoing low-grade inflammation over the course of multiple years, particularly when coupled with significant hormonal fluctuations during perimenopause and menopause, the tissues and muscle can become thinner and drier — and even more susceptible to inflammatory changes. As a result its important to restore our hormonal balance.

Defect in bladder epithelium: A defect in the bladder lining that allows harmful substances in the urine to come into contact with the bladder wall. The bladder has a specialized natural lining called the epithelium. The epithelium is protected from toxins in the urine by a layer of protein called glycosaminoglycan. In people with IC, this protective layer breaks down, allowing toxins to irritate the bladder wall and cause inflammation of the bladder.

NEUROGENIC

The nerves that carry bladder sensations are inflamed, so pain is caused by events that are not normally painful (such as filling of the bladder). Interstitial Cystitis is sometimes also recognized as a chronic neuroinflammatory disorder affecting the bladder — a complex interrelationship between bladder nerves, the immune system, and the urinary tract. Untreated, IC can lead to scarring or stiffening of the bladder walls as well as an inability to hold much fluid in your bladder.

Glomerulations, which are identified as hemorrhages in the mucosal lining of the bladder, and can also develop star-shaped sores called Hunner's ulcers, this is seldom seen in clinical practice.

INFECTIOUS

Although no causative infective agent has been found in the urine of people with IC, an unidentified infectious agent may be the cause.

Injury and chemicals: Urine itself can be an irritant in the urinary tract, mainly if tissues were previously damaged from other primary causes. Urine will change as the diet changes. The urine of people with IC contains a substance known as antiproliferative-factor or APF. APF appears to block the development of cells in the bladder lining. APF inhibits the normal growth of bladder wall cells, making it problematic for your bladder to repair itself if scarred.

This leads scientists to think that some people are predisposed to get Interstitial Cystitis after an injury such as spinal cord trauma, pelvic floor muscle dysfunction, Bladder over distention, damage to pelvic nerves.

Overall different processes occur in different groups of people with IC. It is also likely that different processes may affect each other, for example, a defect in the bladder epithelium may start the inflammation and stimulate mast cells to release histamine.

SYMPTOMS OF IC

Symptoms of Interstitial Cystitis vary from individual to individual. Interstitial Cystitis can affect women and men, even though it is more prevalent in women. Some people may have only a mild sense of urgency while others have multiple symptoms including pain. IC is often diagnosed after other conditions have been ruled out. On average, people with IC experience symptoms for four years before the condition is diagnosed.

Usually the symptoms starts with urgency, then overtime it leads to pain during urination.

PAINFUL URINATION AND/OR BLADDER PAIN

Some have gradual pain when they urinate. Others have pain AFTER they urinate. Others have excruciating pain even if they are not urinating.

- ➢ Pain that worsens during menstruation in women

- ➢ Pain ranging from mild to intense in the bladder and surrounding pelvic region and perineum -- the area between the anus and vagina in women and the anus and scrotum in men.

- ➢ You may experience bladder pressure, bladder pain and sometimes pelvic pain.

- ➢ Intermittent Pain: Pain may come and go, it may be in remission for days, weeks and then it may flares up again for day or weeks. You could also have this ongoing pain in your bladder/urethra.

- ➢ People with IC may have bladder pain that gets worse as the bladder fills. Some people feel the pain in other areas besides the bladder. The pain may be felt in the lower abdomen, lower back, urethra, or the pelvic or perineal area. Men may feel pain in the scrotum, testicles, or penis. Women may experience pain in the vulva or vagina. The pain may be continuous or intermittent.

SEXUAL DIFFICULTIES

Women may have pain during intercourse, and men may have painful orgasm. Painful sexual intercourse in women-imagine scraping on inflamed urethra.

FREQUENT NEED TO URINATE

In extreme cases it could range up to 60 times a day. For most, they need to urinate more often than they did when they were younger. A person with good health on average urinates seven times a day and does not have to get up at night to urinate. A person with IC urinates frequently, both during the day and night. In early or very mild cases, frequency is sometimes the only symptom.

OTHER BLADDER RELATED SYMPTOMS

As frequency becomes more severe, it leads to urgency. As this progresses patient may feel the need to urinate even if only small amounts of urine passes.

In some urgency may also be accompanied by pain, pressure, or spasms. Others may feel a constant urge to urinate that never goes away, even right after urinating.

Pain or discomfort in the scrotum or penis in men maybe present.

Microscopic blood in urine (however this should always warrant trip to doctor and more testing-i.e. to rule out bladder cancer)

Weak flow, and small quantity may also be present and at time urinary incontinence (leakage).

NON-BLADDER RELATED SYMPTOMS

- Digestive problems (IBS, GERD, Constipation, Diarrhea)
- Fibromyalgia/Chronic exhaustion
- Muscular pain
- Migraine headache
- Allergies
- Sleep difficulties
- Depression

Whatever the symptoms may be, however severe, IC, if left untreated can have a long-lasting, debilitating impact on the quality of life.

CHAPTER 3

WHAT ARE MY OPTIONS?

DIET! DIET! DIET!

This is the first thing you must do!!!

The most promising self-care treatment relevant to RDs is diet modification.

A 2004 ICA online survey found 92% of IC patient respondents reported that certain foods and beverages made their symptoms worse, with more than 84% of respondents stating they got some symptom relief from changing their diet.

Then in July 2007, formative research on IC and diet was published in The Journal of Urology, which listed the top trigger foods for IC.

In 2011, the American Urological Association published guidelines that specifically recommended diet modification as one of the first-line of self-care therapies for newly diagnosed IC patients and RDs.

MODIFY YOUR DIET

While there is no evidence that any specific foods *cause* IC, certain studies have reported that up to 90% of patients expressed symptom exacerbation due to certain food, beverage, and dietary supplements. Some people find that certain foods will trigger a flare-up of symptoms. Keeping a food diary and recording when your symptoms flare can help you identify foods that may cause your symptoms to get worse. For 24 hours (or more), jot down what you eat and drink (and smoke), how often you experience the urge to urinate, the level of your pain intensity, and how relieved your bladder feels after urination. You are then able to take your bladder diary with you any time you visit your healthcare practitioner to assist in figuring out patterns and whether or not you could have IC or not. This is one of the only ways for you to see the associations that may not have been seen otherwise. There are many apps available now that do the same. However you will be surprised what you are missing when you don't write it down.

UNDERSTAND YOUR TRIGGERS

See the section above on common Interstitial Cystitis triggers and learn what you can modify in your diet to lessen your symptoms. Everyone is different and has different triggers.

Follow an IC/alkaline diet. Actively managing the acid–alkaline balance in your body can help all urinary disorders, and lessen your discomfort (more on this later). It has also helped women cut down on the foods that cause other inflammatory issues in their bodies.

ELIMINATION DIET

All food items do not affect all people with IC in the same way. Therefore, each person should find out which food item makes one's symptoms worse. This can be done by trying an "elimination diet." On an elimination diet, one needs to stop eating all food items that can make symptoms worse. If symptoms improve on the elimination diet, the food item that was irritating the bladder needs to be identified. This can be done by introducing one food item at a time into the diet. If the addition of the food item does not worsen symptoms, it can be added to the regular diet. In this manner, one can identify the food item that makes symptoms worse and thus avoid it. Eliminating or reducing foods in your diet that are potential bladder irritants may help to relieve the discomfort of Interstitial Cystitis. If you think certain foods may irritate your bladder, try eliminating them from your diet. Reintroduce them one at a time and pay attention to which, if any, affect your symptoms. Keep a daily log.

There is a lot of evidence that this alone can improve your symptoms significantly. However start out slowly, by eliminating few items first and then increase them slowly. Don't try to do too much all at once, this could deter you completely. As mentioned before, food that maybe fine for one person may cause flares in others. It's best to create charts and next to each food item, list date/time you ate it, and how your body reacted to it. Don't forget that it's not just the food, but ingredients in the food that may be causing flares. You can also ask your doctor to recommend a good nutritionist; however most of this can be done by yourself, if you are disciplined.

FOODS THAT HAVE BEEN IMPLICATED IN AGGRAVATING SYMPTOMS OF INTERSTITIAL CYSTITIS ARE THE FOLLOWING

Even though your body may react differently to certain foods, there are still foods that are widely known to be safe and foods that are believed to cause flares. Here are the some of the foods that the Interstitial Cystitis Network calls "the most problematic" because they trigger the most symptoms in most people. These top offenders are an excellent place to start:

These <u>include tomatoes, spices, alcohol, chocolate, caffeinated and citrus beverages, and high-acid foods</u>.

Common bladder irritants — known as the "four Cs" — include: carbonated beverages, caffeine in all forms (including chocolate), citrus products and food containing high concentrations of vitamin C. Also pickled foods and artificial sweeteners may also aggravate symptoms in some people.

Coffee

The acid and caffeine in coffee can cause intense irritation and discomfort. Additionally, caffeine acts as a diuretic. Therefore lowering your coffee consumption to 12 oz. or perhaps much less per day really is a wise decision – in fact, a lot of women with IC should completely eliminate coffee to feel significantly greater pain relief.

Tea

Black teas and even decaffeinated teas can spark inflammation in your bladder. Everyone is different so just trying this for a few days may bring great relief. Green teas and some herbal teas also have a tendency to have a certain level of acidity.

Cranberry and other acidic fruit juices

Cranberry juice is actually frequently recommended for the treatment of urinary tract infections, but an IC bladder is extremely irritated from the level of acidity in cranberry juice. So if juice is a must for you, try less acidic varieties like pear, apple, and blueberry. Pear juices and pear sweeteners are considered your safest bet.

Soda including diet soda

Your average diet soda contains four major bladder irritants in one shiny can: acidic carbonation, citric and phosphoric acids, caffeine, and artificial sweeteners. In case you absolutely need to have a soda, we recommend a non-diet, non-caffeinated root beer, and diluting it with ice cubes or water is certainly a lot better.

Tomatoes

Though they're full of so many good things, tomatoes are also high in potassium, and are highly acidic, too. For tomato-lovers, low-acid varieties might be substituted as an occasional treat.

Artificial food (i.e. aspartame), colorings (dyes) and flavorings

Food colorings happen to be incredibly common in food (even several health foods) in addition to the majority of over-the-counter multivitamins and prescription medications.

Foods that promote yeast

Sugar, vinegar, yeast, malt and other foods can cause yeast overgrowth. You may want to follow a yeast-free, sugar-free diet — many of the women we see with IC symptoms are found to have systemic yeast, but once the yeast overgrowth is resolved, the IC symptoms abate.

Tobacco

Smoking and tobacco use is another trigger. Tobacco is a common trigger because it constricts the bladder's blood vessels, making it harder for our bodies to naturally cleanse inflammatory substances from the bladder tissues.

Gluten

This problematic, inflammatory protein is found naturally in grains and also in several other foods through additives and contamination. Sometimes diagnosis isn't really done properly and you may be intolerant to gluten, even though you may not have celiac disease.

Certain nutrients

A number of patients truly have allergies or severe sensitivities to certain nutrients — which is why you may read advice recommending that patients with IC discontinue multivitamins.

What about vitamin C? Vitamin C creates your pee to become more acidic! This is precisely the reason you should avoid most carbonated soda drink. The pH will drop making your body more acidic. Think of pouring some acid over a scrape or inflamed skin. This is what you are doing. Your bladder is already inflamed! It is not vitamin C alone, but the supplement you take is probably acidic. Vitamin C is great immune system fighter, but if you are suffering from being more acid-avoid vitamin C.

Once you learn what foods set you off, you can begin to create a list of your trigger foods. Once you feel a lot better – which frequently will happen in just a week or two – experiment with just how much of each and every food your body definitely will process comfortably. The initial dietary changes are about calming down the bladder. Once you have gotten a relief from the symptoms you can begin to focus on healing the bladder lining. For example, changing to a more alkalizing diet has tremendous overall health benefits for your body, aside from just reducing your acidic state.

ON THE OTHER HAND, FOODS THAT HAVE BEEN IDENTIFIED AS LEAST BOTHERSOME OR "SAFE" TO PATIENTS ARE

If you don't know where to start with diet options, consider these foods first, they have been known to be least bothersome to patients.

- Milk/Cottage cheese/Yogurt and dairy –Monitor your gastro condition, and again too much dairy products increase acidic condition. However fermented products may yield beneficial from probiotics.
- Bananas-Make sure you are not sensitive to K+
- Fruits (are great in vitamins/minerals, however they are high in sugar so be careful. Especially avoid dry fruits due to their sugar content)
  - Blueberries
  - Melon

- ➢ Vegetables – Green vegetables encouraged due to their alkalizing properties, however most vegetable should be ok.

    - o Carrots
    - o Broccoli
    - o Mushrooms
    - o Peas

- ➢ Grains-whole wheat, white wheat may be hard to tolerate. Instead try:

    - o Millet
    - o Quinoa
    - o Buckwheat
    - o Rice

- ➢ Meat-Most meats are acidic, if you are working on alkalizing diet, avoid meat. Otherwise some white meat should be fine:

    - o Chicken
    - o Fish
    - o Egss

- Water-Alkalized water! If you don't know if the water you are having is alkalized, you can call the manufacturer. You can also get your water from alkalizing water store. If nothing else, you can also simply add green powder or cucumber/lemon to your water to make it more alkalized. Sometimes filtered water helps, since lot of tap water maybe chlorinated. Hydrate! Hydrate! Hydrate! Drink water! It is vital to stay hydrated; water helps cleanse away viruses in your body and places you on the right track to restoration. It is better to have a steady flow of water throughout the day then having a large quantity all at once and then not having any for hours. I know this is hard since with IC you have the urgency and pain, but you do need to get your daily water intake. Tap water may be fine, however you do want to stay a little alkaline and investigate a little into the amount of fluoride and chlorine that is placed in it as this maybe killing good bacteria and eventually causing some imbalance in your gut. Especially if you are taking probiotics, chlorine is a disinfectant and may be counterproductive if you are taking probiotics with chlorinated water. I recommend you consume in ounces half your body weight. If you weigh 200lbs, consume 100 ounce of water a day, remember you want to stay hydrated throughout the day so don't just drink big jugs twice a day and forget about it.

➢ Tea-chamomile and peppermint tea are best

SUPPLEMENTING YOUR DIET WITH PROBIOTICS

"Good bacteria", "Beneficial bacteria", "Gut flora" are great for so many reasons. However personally I believe there are so many probiotics on the market that are useless. They are not potent and are a waste of money. For instance, did you know that the number of probiotics that you are actually consuming is far less than what's indicated on the bottle label? Probiotics manufacturers are only required to place the number of probiotics at time of manufacturing. Most of these bacteria die by the time you consume them. They die during transport, they die on shelves at your supermarket, and even the ones that are supposedly inside a refrigeration unit may not always have been refrigerated during the entire shipping process and could be dead and thus not viable.

If you have found a good source, stick to it-this will also take some time. However over the long term this could get expensive. If you are consuming probiotics and are not feeling better or they are too expensive for you; I suggest you make your own probiotics. I recommend <u>purchasing kefir grains and making your own kefir</u>. You will literally save thousands of dollars. You are also guaranteed to consume a large quantity of fresh, thriving bacteria, since for milk to ferment you know the bacteria must be present. It is important to purchase high quality kefir grains and it is also important that you follow strict guidelines on how to make your first few batches until your live cultures are striving. There are many books on amazon that show you a <u>step-by-step guide on how to make kefir</u>.

ALKALIZE

Acidosis or the accumulation of acidic wastes throughout the body maybe leading to general malaise and triggering some IC symptoms.

Acid in stomach helps us to digest our food. However it is the waste created after metabolizing food within our cells and tissues that could be hampering our health. Acid is a natural by-product of the combustion of digestion and our system is normally equipped to neutralize this acid-when a balanced diet is eaten. However, today's diet tends to be more processed and more acidic with the intake of high protein and/or high sugar foods, including simple carbohydrates.

Since your blood pH must remain the same, the rest of the body does what is necessary to insure blood pH stability. One thing that happens when the body is overloaded with acid and its byproducts is that in an effort to maintain stability of blood pH at all costs, the body will "grab" for the handiest alkalizing source which unfortunately may be your bones- not the most ideal choice as an alkalizing agent.

While an alkaline diet alone will not completely cure you of serious diseases, it's worth notating that many people saw a decrease in IC symptoms after having followed an alkalizing, anti-inflammatory diet by avoiding certain trigger foods such as eliminating caffeine, alcohol and smoking.

Remember people will often try to sell you alkalizing products. However you don't need much to alkalizing except changing your diet to include foods that are alkalizing.

The cheapest, most effective and simplest way to alkalize your body is bye eating green vegetables!

INTERSTITIAL CYSTITIS CURE

ALKALIZING FOODS
ALKALIZING VEGETABLES

Asparagus	Kiwi	Seaweed
Barley Grass	Kohlrabi	Spinach
Beets	Lettuce	Spirulina
Broccoli	Mushrooms	Sprouts
Brussel sprouts	Mustard Greens	Squashes
Cabbage	Dulce	Watercress
Carrot	Dandelions	Wheat Grass
Cauliflower	Edible Flowers	Wild Greens
*Celery (	Nightshade Veggies	**ORIENTAL VEGETABLES**
Chard	Onions	Maitake
Chlorella	Parsnips (high glycemic)	Daikon
Collard Greens	Parsley	Dandelion Root
Cucumber	Peas	Shitake
Eggplant	Peppers	Kombu
Fermented Veggies	Pumpkin	Reishi
Garlic	Rutabaga	Nori
Kale	Sea Veggies	Umeboshi
		Wakame

*Celery plant seeds also act as a diuretic, due mainly to one of the elements of celery oil, butylphthalide. Eating a few celery plant seeds can help increase the development of pee. If you want to get some more liquid, create celery seeds water.)
Most vegetables are by nature alkalizing

ALKALIZING FRUITS

Apple	All Berries
Apricot	Tangerine
Avocado	Tomato
Banana (high glycemic)	Tropical Fruits
Cantaloupe	Watermelon
Cherries	
Currants	Be aware of high sugar content in most fruits, this alone can trigger IC symptoms!
Coconut water	
Dates/Figs	
Grapes	
Grapefruit	
Lime	
Honeydew Melon	
Nectarine	
Orange	
Lemon	
Peach	
Pear	
Pineapple	

INTERSTITIAL CYSTITIS CURE

ALKALIZING PROTEIN	OTHER	SWEETENERS
Eggs	Apple Cider Vinegar	Stevia
Whey Protein Powder	Bee Pollen	
Cottage Cheese	Lecithin Granules	SPICES/SEASONINGS
Chicken Breast	Probiotic Cultures	Cinnamon
Yogurt	Green Juices	Curry
Almonds	Veggies Juices	Ginger
Chestnuts	Fresh Fruit Juice	Mustard
Tofu (fermented)	Organic Milk (unpasteurized)	Chili Pepper
Flax Seeds	Mineral Water	Sea Salt
Pumpkin Seeds	Alkaline Antioxidant Water	Miso
Tempeh (fermented)	Green Tea	Tamari
Squash Seeds	Herbal Tea	All Herbs
Sunflower Seeds	Dandelion Tea	
Millet	Ginseng Tea	
Sprouted Seeds	Banchi Tea	
Nuts	Kombucha	
Most meat/protein by nature is acidic. You may be able to get away with having moderate amount of these- Proceed with caution		

ACIDIFYING FOODS

FATS & OILS	Corn	Brazil Nuts
Avocado Oil	Oats (rolled)	Peanuts
Canola Oil	Quinoa	Peanut Butter
Corn Oil	Rice (all)	Pecans
Hemp Seed Oil	Rye	Tahini
Flax Oil	Spelt	Walnuts
Lard	Kamut	
Olive Oil	Wheat	ANIMAL PROTEIN
Safflower Oil	Hemp Seed Flour	Beef
Sesame Oil		Carp
Sunflower Oil	DAIRY	Clams
	Cheese, Cow	Fish
FRUITS	Cheese, Goat	Lamb
Cranberries	Cheese, Processed	Lobster
	Cheese, Sheep	Mussels
GRAINS	Milk	Oyster
Rice Cakes	Butter	Pork
Wheat Cakes		Rabbit
Amaranth	NUTS & BUTTERS	Salmon
Barley	Cashews	Shrimp
Buckwheat		

INTERSTITIAL CYSTITIS CURE

ACIDIFYING FOODS

ANIMAL PROTEIN CON'T	Herbicides
Scallops	
Tuna	**ALCOHOL**
Turkey	Beer
Venison	Spirits
	Hard Liquor
PASTA (WHITE)	Wine
Noodles	
Macaroni	**BEANS & LEGUMES**
Spaghetti	Black Beans
	Chick Peas
OTHER	Green Peas
Distilled Vinegar	Kidney Beans
Wheat Germ	Lentils
Potatoes	Lima Beans
	Pinto Beans
DRUGS & CHEMICALS	Red Beans
Chemicals	Soy Beans
Drugs, Medicinal	Soy Milk
Drugs, Psychedelic	White Beans
Pesticides	Rice Milk
	Almond Milk

CHAPTER 4

NOT GETTING BETTER WITH IC DIET, WHY???

I'm following the IC diet….why don't I feel better? There are thousands of food options out there, especially as you add spices, oil and other micronutrients that play major role in flare up. The above list has been designed as a starting point and is not all inclusive. These are list of common food that have been researched or known to be "safe" and not cause flare up.

However that does not mean you will not exhibit symptoms from eating those foods. It only means majority of people have not exhibited symptoms from these and this maybe a good starting point.

So, what in your diet is causing your flare up and why is it so hard to pinpoint? Many patients are diagnosed with having IC, but the source may have nothing to do with a urinary or bladder issue. A high percentage of IC patients tends to be fatigued, have digestive issues, are sensitive to acidic condition, and/or are intolerant to gluten; they have also been known to have different allergies, weak immune system, etc.… Therefore you need to figure out what is the source of your ailment? Are you digestive issue causing IC? If you improve your digestion will this get rid of your IC symptoms? Is there overgrowth of candida, and if you were to control your sugar, does this get rid of your IC symptoms? Is your body too acidic and if you were to alkalize your body, does this magically rid your IC symptoms? This is where you really need a diary or good monitoring device to weed out the problematic food.

For example: Dairy products (cheese, milk, ice cream, yogurt) could be bad if you are having gastrointestinal issues or are lactose intolerant or having a hard time digesting food. Probiotics found in yogurt, kefir, cottage cheese and other dairy products are great if you have candida or other fungal overgrowths or digestive imbalance, but not if you are lactose intolerant. Your symptoms may only flare up when you eat certain grains, perhaps you are sensitive to gluten (the protein found in grains). Meat could be fine if you are gluten intolerant, but if you are trying to alkalize it maybe bad as you are increasing acidic environment. Greens could be great for alkalizing but if you are having loose stool and over eating fiber then this could cause other digestive issues. Fruits for example are great for vitamins/minerals, have beneficial fiber, however they are high in sugar.

Are you confused yet? All these problems could be crisscrossing. Diet sounds easy compared to other methods but <u>requires great discipline</u>. Even when you have great discipline it requires good book keeping. This is why one answer doesn't work for everyone. **Someone who tells you eat lots of fruits or eat lots of protein, eat a lot of yogurt, avoid all grains, go on this diet and that diet, and buy this supplement and the other, etc., maybe trying to sell you something or telling you only half-truth!** The only real way to monitor this is to keep good book keeping. None of this will happen overnight. You didn't develop IC overnight and you won't lose it overnight. Like everything else it's what you do every day that makes a difference not what you do once in a while. So stick to it. Give it adequate time for something to work. It is very important to monitor in detail everything that is going into your mouth.

I would recommend you create a food log, identifying everything you eat, the time you eat, time you feel pain, intensity of the pain, (1-10 scale or three type scale: good, medium, and bad). In the beginning start with plain/simple foods (food that doesn't have too many ingredients, bland, not overly processed). For every food you do well with –put them into your temporary safe list (try this food again in a week) do this 3 times before you put it on your permanent safe list. Slowly and slowly you will increase your safe list, and you can start picking foods off that without having flares. At times you will find yourself eating food that once had no flare but the second time you ate it, it caused intense pain. First make sure you didn't add other ingredients to it, start to look at other factors (are you dehydrated, stress level, spicy food eaten earlier, too much coffee or acidic conditions prior to eating that meal, etc....) Make sure you indicate this in your journal. There may be food that you eat that may not cause flares right away but after a day or two or even week. So keep in mind something you at a week ago. This will be very difficult in the beginning but you will soon see a trend of food that are just not causing any flare up. Once you have a list know you can always go to these foods. Again first begin with basic food type, you can even pick some off the suggested food above, until you get your own safe list. (i.e. potato, plain bread, plain ice cream, etc....) This will be the most difficult at first since you already don't have a proven safe list made up. Remember the more detailed in your journal the more information you have to assess. Also note the quantity of food you are consuming, some food will cause flare up even if you have very little, others you can tolerate in larger amounts but may eventually cause flare ups. There are many useful food tracking apps that can help you document this.

CHAPTER 5

EASE THE PAIN ALKALIZE ON THE SPOT

In a 2011 study, calcium glycerophosphate and sodium bicarbonate showed a trend toward improvement of symptoms.

Drink this

If you are in pain! Alkalize on the spot by taking organic aloe-Vera with a spoon of baking soda or eno. Basically baking soda will alkalize your system at once. It has high pH and is more alkaline. This should help you on the spot! You can take this every 3hrs or so, however keep in mind don't make this a dietary habit, there are other issues associated with regular use of baking soda.

Once the pain is manageable you can continue drinking aloe vera with two spoons of lemon juice. You can also follow this as your daily morning routine. First thing in the morning have a glass of water with a little lemon juice in it. Lemon juice is acidic but in your body it becomes alkaline. Some suggest mixing lemon juice and baking soda with water (However I haven't gotten a clear answer on this, because lemon juice is acidic it reacts with baking soda alkaline and don't know if the liquid then neutralizes, before you ingest it).

Take a glass of this and then get another glass and sip on it for the next 3 hours. Wait a couple of hours and drink another glass. This will alkalize you quickly, and then try following the above diet.

SUPPLEMENTS

"AZO bladder" tablet may provide short term relief, however note your urine color may change and it may provide staining of clothes. AZO bladder pain tablet over the counter-look into this to manager your bladder pain.

Prelief may also help you for quick temporary relief if you are suffering from acidic environment. Similar to other antacids, like Tums that help with upper GI, Prelief is said to help with lower urinary by eliminating acid from food you eat.

Butterbur tablets are also known to help during flare ups.

Quercetin is an anti-inflammatory and may also help with your pain symptoms. Quercetin, is an antioxidant in the flavonol group with marked anti-inflammatory actions. It is also very effective in decreasing systemic allergic responses. Quercetin-containing supplements are exceptionally well tolerated and are reported to provide considerable symptomatic improvement in patients with IC.

Neem/Licorice/Asparagus Tablet- You may also want to take asparagus extract, neem tablets or even licorice root tea/capsules, all of which may help during a flare up episode.

Turmeric is a fabulous anti-inflammatory agent along with boswellia.

Omega-3s have long been known for their ability to decrease systemic inflammation in the tissue and membranes.

Digestive enzymes- Most in my opinion are marketing scams, but you can always try them to see if you feel any different from taking them. If you do try them, give it an adequate amount of time to see if consuming it makes a different. If you want a cheaper alternative try consuming some sauerkraut with every meal for a week and see if this makes a difference.

Probiotics also help restore normal flora and lessen inflammation, plus help to combat systemic yeast triggers. However I wouldn't recommend probiotics for immediate relief. It takes time to normalize gut flora. I would definitely consider them for overall plan, but not necessarily for quick immediate relief.

An alternative to probiotics is kefir. Here's why: The probiotic numbers you see on the bottle are probiotics that were tested at the time of manufacturing. Therefore the actual probiotics in those bottles may be next to nil. Numbers of probiotics you see on the probiotics bottles are not the number of live probiotics that you are consuming!!

If you are on a probiotic and can feel the difference keep it up. However if you have given few a try and are not seeing the results it's time to make your own probiotics/Kefir from grains!

This is why I recommend <u>making your own probiotics</u> and consuming fresh batches daily. This way you take out all the variables, all the marketing gimmicks and you know what you are getting.

DON'T FALL FOR DIET SCAMS

Be wary of any alkaline diet resource that argues that the only way to follow the diet properly is to buy specially-formulated (usually expensive) foods. These are, almost without exception, scams. A simple look at the list of ingredients above should be enough to reveal that it's possible to get all of the foods you need to follow an alkaline diet at your normal grocery store, so don't waste your money on dubious alternatives. Rule of thumb is if it's green vegetables it's probably alkaline.

SHOULD I PEE OFTEN OR HOLD IT IN?

People with IC may be able to reduce urinary frequency by using bladder-training techniques. They are advised to progressively increase the voiding (emptying the bladder) interval over the course of weeks to months by using relaxation techniques and distractions. A diary can help track the progress. Whenever you vacate your bladder — even if it's just a little bit — you rid some of the bacterias. This is great if you are suffering from UTI or have an infection. However if you are continuing to go to the restroom with very little pee coming out, then over time you are conditioning your bladder to go to the bathroom often. You may want to think about training your bladder; if you are home you can slowly train your bladder not to go to the bathroom at first urgency. Slowly work to train your bladder longer and longer. Bladder training involves timed urination — going to the toilet according to the clock rather than waiting for the need to go. You start by urinating at set intervals, such as every half-hour — whether you have to go or not. Then you gradually wait longer between bathroom visits. During bladder training, you may learn to control urinary urges by using relaxation techniques, such as breathing slowly and deeply or distracting yourself with another activity. How do you know bladder Training is working? You will want to measure how much are you peeing, are you slowly increasing amount of pee when you void? This may be another item you write in your journal, this way you can see if bladder training is actually working. Over time this will also train your bladder muscles.

PHYSICAL THERAPY

Try physical therapy. Most people with IC also have severe pelvic floor dysfunction, a condition in which the muscles of the pelvic floor do not relax enough to allow easy urination. They also may have alignment issues as well. Physical therapy to rehabilitate the pelvic floor is very helpful in easing the pain of IC, as is bladder "retraining" to gradually expand the time between trips to the bathroom. And a technique called myofascial tissue manipulation and polarity therapy shows promise for reducing IC symptoms.

SMOKING/TOBACCO

If you smoke, stop. Smoking may worsen any painful condition, and smoking contributes to bladder cancer. Many people with IC have reported that smoking makes their symptoms worse. Quitting smoking will not only provide symptomatic relief to people with IC but will also decrease the risk of developing bladder cancer, because smoking is a known cause of bladder cancer. Smoking cessation will also decrease the incidence of heart disease, hypertension, stroke, peripheral vascular disease, and lung cancer.

EXERCISE

Ok you didn't pay for this book to get on some exercise program. So I won't make it lengthy-but **it is very important**!!! I recommend at least 30 minutes a day, enough to get your heart rate up. The endorphins that kick in after exercising actually helps the immune system and ultimately fight of ailments. Easy stretching exercises such as yoga and pilates may help reduce your Interstitial Cystitis symptoms. This will add flexibility to your pelvic region. If you are hesitant or not in shape for a hard gut-wrenching exercise, do yoga or pilates. Heart pounding, cardio exercise benefits you in a completely different way over slower, flexible, mind-calming exercises that effects the body differently.

MEDITATE

Many people also find that symptoms become worse if they have stress (either physical or mental stress). In women, symptoms may vary with the menstrual cycle; symptoms often get worse during periods. As you've heard many times, stress is the root cause of many physical and mental ailments. Anything that calms your nerves down-including the ones that are making you go pee often would be a plus. Do you ever have to go pee when you are nervous or have butteflies? Well what if you are always insecure, scared, have your nerves on edge all of the time? Try calming your nerves and reducing stress by learning simple meditation techniques such as visualization or guided imagery. This type of therapy employs visualization and direct suggestions using imagery to help you imagine healing, with the hope that the body will follow the mind's suggestions.

USE HEAT/BATH IN LAVENDER OR EPSOM SALT

When IC symptoms flare up and you experience the swelling and discomfort causing continuous, irritating discomfort, try a warm water bath with either Epsom salt or lavender oil over your bladder which may bring you some comfort.

ACUPUNCTURE

During an acupuncture session, a practitioner places numerous thin needles in your skin at specific points on your body. According to traditional Chinese medicine, precisely placed acupuncture needles relieve pain and other symptoms by rebalancing the flow of life energy. Western medical practitioners tend to believe that acupuncture boosts the activity of your body's natural painkillers. If you are going to do acupuncture I suggest you stick to it for 2-3 months, it takes time for your body to shift.

If you cannot find other causes for your allergic reaction to foods, consider

NAET

NAET is an allergy elimination technique that has helped some people overcome problematic allergies and sensitivities. However it has not proven successful for everyone, including myself.

Alternative theories include the mechanism of "cross-talk," or the idea that stimuli from one organ can lead to changes in another organ by integrated sensory pathways. In other words, stimulation of the bowel by certain dietary substances can modulate pelvic pain in Interstitial Cystitis/bladder pain syndrome.

CHAPTER 6

MEDICAL ROUTE

WHAT'S WRONG WITH IC PATIENTS MEDICALLY SPEAKING?

The medical theory is that (K+) excreted by the kidneys in high concentration irritates and damages the bladder because the bladder lining (epithelium) is deficient in its protective layer of mucus (called the glycosoaminoglycan or GAG layer). When this layer gets depleted your bladder is susceptible to irritation. A leak in the epithelium may allow toxic substances in urine to irritate your bladder wall. Treatment is to fix the GAG layer, which will coat the bladder wall and allow for normal function of the bladder.

POTASSIUM SENSITIVITY TEST

Potassium sensitivity test is conducted for this reason. In this test, the urinary bladder is filled with either potassium solution or water, and pain and/or urgency scores are compared. A person who has IC feels more pain and/or urgency when the bladder is filled with the potassium solution than when the bladder is filled with water. However, people with normal bladders cannot tell the difference between the two solutions.

It is approximated that about one-quarter of individuals have bladder or pelvic issues due to lack GAG. Currently a drug called "Elmiron" is mostly prescribed for IC. This drug takes months before it can be effective. This is not an overnight cure drug, and it will not ease your flares. Urologist also prescribe this when they just run out of options on what could be causing IC. Therefore it is not a positive diagnosis, but it is based on ruling other things out, unless your doctors would consider doing "Potassium sensitivity test". In this test, your doctor places two solutions — water and potassium chloride — into your bladder, one at a time. You're asked to rate on a scale of 0 to 5 the pain and urgency you feel after each solution is instilled. If you feel noticeably more pain or urgency with the potassium solution than with the water, your doctor may diagnose interstitial cystitis. People with normal bladders can't tell the difference between the two solutions.

DOCTOR'S VISIT

On your visit to the doctor you can discuss the volume of fluids you drink and the volume of urine you pass. Foods that trigger symptoms, time of day, how often you get up to go to the bathroom at night, do spicy food trigger it more, etc…

You may also request to get your pelvic exam done, your doctor examines your external genitals, vagina and cervix and feels your abdomen to assess your internal pelvic organs. Your doctor may also examine your anus and rectum.

Urine test

A sample of your urine will be analyzed for evidence of a urinary tract infection. Urine culture: This test can be used to identify the organisms that cause urinary tract infections. For this exam, a midstream specimen of urine is obtained in a sterile container after the genital area is washed. In people with IC, the urine is sterile and no bacterial growth is obtained.

Antibiotics

If you have an infection you will be prescribed antibiotics. This will kill the bacteria and VIOLA!!! However if you have been diagnosed with IC, you probably already know you don't have an infection. You also probably have already tried doses of antibiotics to no avail. FOR MEN: SOME MEN WILL HAVE IC SYMPTOMS FOR YEARS BUT IT IS NOT A BLADDER ISSUE. IT IS "PROSTATITS". THIS GOES UNDER THE RADAR, MANY TIMES. A WEEK OR TWO OF ANTIBIOTICS WILL NOT CURE THIS. YOU WILL NEED A MONTH OR MORE OF ANTIBIOTICS! This is inflammation of your prostate gland. This may reoccur over the years, whenever your immune system takes a dive. Please ask your doctor about this!

MRI

Next step the doctor probably check your kidney. If kidneys are functioning fine and you don't have any kidney stones.

Cystoscopy

With cystoscopy, your doctor inserts a thin tube with a tiny camera (cystoscope) through the urethra, which allows your doctor to see the lining of your bladder. Along with cystoscopy, your doctor may inject liquid into your bladder to measure your bladder capacity. Your doctor may perform this procedure, known as hydrodistention, after you've been numbed with an anesthetic medication to make you more comfortable. Cystoscopy with distention of the bladder: If no infectious agent is identified in the urine, cystoscopy is performed. In this procedure, the health-care provider uses a cystoscope (a hollow tube with a light source) to see the inside of the bladder. The bladder wall is stretched by filling it with liquid or gas. This procedure may be performed under anesthesia because it may be painful. People with IC may have pinpoint hemorrhages, called glomerulations, in the bladder wall and/or ulcers (an open sore in the lining of the bladder), which can be viewed during the procedure.

Biopsy

During cystoscopy under anesthesia, your doctor may remove a sample of tissue (biopsy) from the bladder and the urethra for examination under a microscope. This is to check for bladder cancer and other rare causes of bladder pain. This test helps to rule out bladder cancer.

ORAL MEDICATIONS

Drugs should be considered after conservative measures have failed to provide substantial improvement in symptoms.

Oral medications may improve the signs and symptoms of interstitial cystitis.

Over the counter

There are nonsteroidal anti-inflammatory drugs, such as ibuprofen (Advil, Motrin IB, others) or naproxen (Aleve), to relieve pain.

Antihistamines:

Antihistamines can be helpful in treating IC. Hydroxyzine (Atarax, Vistaril, 25-75 mg at bedtime), loratadine, Claritin, cimetidine (Tagamet, 300 mg twice daily) are the only antihistaminics that have been specifically used for the treatment of people with IC. They may reduce urinary urgency and frequency and relieve other symptoms. Hydroxyzine is an H1 histamine receptor blocker that may inhibit mast cell secretion and may suppress histamine activity in the subcortical region of the central nervous system (CNS). The main side effect of hydroxyzine is sedation, which is actually a benefit because it helps the person with IC to sleep better at night and get up to urinate less frequently.

Anticholinergics and antimuscarinics are the mainstay therapy for overactive bladder, urgency, and urge incontinence. They have a central role in IC. Tolteradine (Detrol), oxybutynin (Ditropan), and others are used extensively with good results and few side effects. High doses may be required, and combination therapy may be effective.

Antidepressants

Tricyclic antidepressants, such as amitriptyline or imipramine (Tofranil) can be used to help relax your bladder and block the pain. Tricyclic antidepressants (amitriptyline [Elavil, 25-75 mg at bedtime], doxepin [Adapin, Sinequan, 75 mg at bedtime], and imipramine [Tofranil, 25 mg three times a day]) are used in people with IC for their pain-relieving effects. They alleviate both the pain and frequency of IC and also help deal with the psychological stress associated with a chronically painful condition. They also cause drowsiness and deepen REM sleep, which helps in decreasing nocturia.

ELmiron

Currently, there's only one medication available that specifically treats IC, <u>Pentosan (ELMIRON)</u> however it only helps 30% to 40% of IC patients. This drug is approved by the Food and Drug Administration specifically for treating interstitial cystitis. How it works is unknown, but it may restore the inner surface of the bladder, which protects the bladder wall from substances in urine that could irritate it. It may take two to four months before you begin to feel pain relief and up to six months to experience a decrease in urinary frequency. Sodium pentosan polysulfate (Elmiron) is the only oral drug approved by the U.S. Food and Drug

Administration (FDA) for the treatment of people with IC. Its mode of action is not entirely understood, but it may act as an antiinflammatory agent. Because it is structurally similar to naturally occurring glucosaminoglycans, it is believed to restore the protective layer on the bladder epithelium. Sodium pentosan polysulfate also has some anticoagulant action, and caution should be used when other anticoagulants are given. The dosage is 100 mg orally three times a day. Clinical studies suggest that maximal effects are not observed until the drug has been taken for at least five to six months. Side effects of sodium pentosan polysulfate include headache, rash, dizziness, diarrhea, dyspepsia, abdominal pain, hair loss (which is reversible), and liver function abnormalities. Pentosan polysulfate sodium is a negatively charged, synthetic sulfated polysaccharide with an affinity for mucosal membranes. It repletes defects in the glycosaminoglycan layer. Adult dosing is 100mg orally 3 times daily. Pentosan polysulfate sodium is a pregnancy category B drug. A following procedure may be considered, but you will have to talk to your doctor. Elmiron or heparin mixed with a local anesthetic (Xylocaine) and alkalinizing agent (sodium bicarbonate) is placed into the empty bladder via a small catheter. Then you wait 30-45 minutes before voiding. This is done three times weekly for two to three weeks while oral medication is instituted. This can help with flares while effect of elmiron kicks in.

For patients who have very severe interstitial cystitis and a variety of otherconditions listed earlier-now being called LUDE or Lower Urinary Dysfunctional Epithelium-they can be taught to self-administer this mixture. Published literature on this program is pending, as these are very new and exciting results from ongoing research.

Aside from drug you may also want to consider the following treatment options:

NERVE STIMULATION TECHNIQUES

Transcutaneous electrical nerve stimulation (TENS).

With TENS, mild electrical pulses relieve pelvic pain and, in some cases, reduce urinary frequency. TENS may work by increasing blood flow to the bladder, strengthening the muscles that help control the bladder or triggering the release of substances that block pain. Electrical wires placed on your lower back or just above your pubic area deliver electrical pulses — the length of time and frequency of therapy depends on what works best for you.

Sacral nerve stimulation

Your sacral nerves are a primary link between the spinal cord and nerves in your bladder. Stimulating these nerves may reduce urinary urgency associated with interstitial cystitis. With sacral nerve stimulation, a thin wire placed near the sacral nerves delivers electrical impulses to your bladder, similar to what a pacemaker does for your heart. If the procedure decreases your symptoms, you may have a permanent device surgically implanted.

Bladder distention

Some people notice a temporary improvement in symptoms after undergoing cystoscopy with bladder distention. Bladder distention is the stretching of the bladder with water or gas. The procedure may be repeated as a treatment if the response is long lasting.

Bladder Drug Instillation (Bladder Wash)

In bladder instillation, your doctor places the prescription medication dimethyl sulfoxide (Rimso-50) into your bladder through a thin, flexible tube (catheter) inserted through the urethra. The solution sometimes is mixed with other medications, such as a local anesthetic, and remains in your bladder for 15 minutes. You urinate to expel the solution.

Dimethyl sulfoxide (DMSO, Rimso-50) is the only drug approved by the FDA for use in bladder instillation. The technique does not require anesthesia, hospitalization, or the use of an operating room. This treatment is given every week or two weeks for six to eight weeks. DMSO is believed to work as an antiinflammatory agent and therefore reduces pain. It may also prevent contractions that cause pain, frequency, and urgency. By the end of the sessions, complete relief of symptoms is often obtained.

If symptoms recur, more treatments can be given. People who are willing to catheterize themselves may be able to self-administer treatments at home. Side effects include a garlic-like body odor in some people. For some people, DMSO instillations can be painful. This can often be relieved by first instilling a local anesthetic into the bladder through a catheter or by mixing the local anesthetic with DMSO. Some clinicians substitute intravesical (instilled in the bladder) heparin for DMSO. Other agents can be added to DMSO making an IC "cocktail." These include corticosteroids, heparin, normal saline (sodium chloride solution), and lidocaine.

A newer approach to bladder instillation uses a solution containing the medications lidocaine, sodium bicarbonate, and either pentosan or heparin. If patients still do not respond, intravesical therapy may be initiated, beginning with weekly dimethyl sulfoxide (DMSO) therapy for 6 courses. Dimethyl sulfoxide (DMSO) provides anti-inflammatory action, membrane penetration, antifungal activity, cryoprotective effects for living cells and tissues, collagen dissolution action, mast cell stimulation, nerve blockade, diuresis, cholinesterase inhibition, vasodilation, and muscle relaxation. It may be combined with heparin, steroids, or bicarbonate. Monthly maintenance DMSO instillations have been advocated by some clinicians in order to prevent flares, although data supporting this approach are lacking.

DMSO

DMSO may be combined with steroids, bicarbonate, and heparin. Intravesical lidocaine may also be added. Some patients with refractory interstitial cystitis symptoms self-catheterize at home and instill a variety of these medications intravesically on an as-needed basis for symptom flares or simply for long-term therapy.

NEW EMERGING STUDIES

In patients who respond poorly to DMSO, intravesical heparin or sodium oxychlorosene (Clorpactin) may be tried. Long-term application of capsaicin, a component of hot pepper, has been associated with the desensitization of C fibers, the unmyelinated nerve fibers known for transmitting pain. Intravesical instillation of capsaicin has been limited in its use in interstitial cystitis because of the sensation of severe burning.

Resiniferatoxin

Resiniferatoxin, a capsaicin analogue, is 100-10,000 times more potent than capsaicin and is not associated with severe burning. However, resiniferatoxin has shown poor effectiveness after single administration, with no significant improvement in symptoms of interstitial cystitis, and side effects of dose-dependent pain and urgency symptoms. A meta-analysis by Guo et al in 2013 showed that no significant improvement was achieved in patients treated with resiniferatoxin in terms of frequency, nocturia, incontinence, or involuntary detrusor contractions.

Hyaluronic Acid

Hyaluronic acid glycosaminoglycan replenishment therapy has yielded moderate results in non–placebo-controlled studies. In a study of weekly instillation of a 50-mL solution of phosphate-buffered solution containing 40 mg of sodium hyaluronate, 85% and 84% of patients reported symptomatic and quality-of-life improvement, respectively, with 50% of patients reporting a lasting effect at 5-year follow-up. Patients in this study had demonstrated abnormal results on a modified potassium sensitivity test. Lower response rates are seen in patients without evidence of a urine-tissue barrier abnormality. Currently, several studies with level 2b evidence support hyaluronic acid instillation. Patients report decreases in visual analog pain scores. Multicenter, randomized trials do not exist, however.

Hydrodistention/Hyaluronic Acid

Patients in whom medical therapy fails may benefit from another bladder hydrodistention if the first hydrodistention was therapeutic. In the rare patient in whom a Hunner ulcer is seen on cystoscopy, cauterization or laser fulguration of the ulcer is recommended.In combination with hydrodistension, hyaluronic acid has been shown to maintain or prolong the effect of hydrodistension in some patients with IC.

Additional smaller studies have shown that both hyaluronic acid and chondroitin sulfate had sustained improvement in symptomatology Unfortunately, other small studies have not been able to support the use of chondroitin sulfate as a monotherapy for IC, despite small improvements in pain scores.

Intravesical bacillus Calmette-Guérin

Intravesical bacillus Calmette-Guérin (BCG) has been hypothesized to suppress inflammation within the bladder. A randomized, placebo-controlled trial in patients with refractory interstitial cystitis revealed borderline statistical significance for global response assessment questioning, as well as most secondary outcome measures, including capacity, pain scores, urgency/frequency symptoms, and interstitial cystitis inventories. Similar to resiniferatoxin, there is currently recommendation against this treatment.

Intravesical liposomes

Experimental therapies include treatment with intravesical liposomes, which are vesicles composed of concentric phospholipid bilayers. These adsorb to cell surfaces and act as a delivery mechanisms for various chemicals. Animal models have shown decreased bladder sensitivity to potassium chloride, and small human studies have shown promising results in reduction of frequency, nocturia, pain, urgency, and O'Leary-Sant scores. While these results are initially promising, large, randomized trials are still lacking.

Hyperbaric Oxygen

Hyperbaric oxygen is also an emerging treatment. As this has been successfully used to treat hemorrhagic cystitis from cyclophosphamide and radiation, it was used in a pilot study in patients with refractory IC/BPS. Seven of 11 patients showed durable improvement in pain scores and urgency symptoms lasing over 2 years. This may also be a useful adjunct to DMSO instillation.

Corticosteroids Silver nitrate

Corticosteroids Silver nitrate is used for its caustic, antiseptic, and astringent qualities. In adults, administer concentrations ranging from 1:5000 to 2% intravesically for 2-10 minutes. Silver nitrate is a pregnancy category C drug.

Sodium oxychlorosene

Sodium oxychlorosene exerts detergent action on bladder mucosa. It is reserved for patients in whom DMSO or silver nitrate instillations fail.

Immunosuppressives Heparin

Polysaccharide glycosaminoglycans may exert a protective effect on the bladder. Heparin has been shown to reduce relapses in patients who respond to DMSO. It is an analogue to the polysaccharide glycosaminoglycan lining of the bladder.

SURGERY

Doctors rarely use surgery to treat Interstitial Cystitis because removing part or all of the bladder doesn't relieve pain and can lead to other complications. People with severe pain or those whose bladders can hold only very small volumes of urine are possible candidates for surgery, but usually only after other treatments have failed. Surgery is usually reserved for patients with ulcers on the bladder. And it's generally seen as a final option after other treatments have failed to work. But doctors often discourage it because some people will still have symptoms after the surgery.

Fulguration

This minimally invasive method involves insertion of instruments through the urethra to burn off ulcers that may be present with interstitial cystitis.

Resection

This is another minimally invasive method that involves insertion of instruments through the urethra to cut around any ulcers.

Bladder augmentation

In this procedure, surgeons remove the damaged portion of the bladder and replace it with a piece of the colon, but the pain still remains and some people need to empty their bladders with a catheter many times.

CONCLUSION

No simple treatment exists to eliminate the signs and symptoms of Interstitial Cystitis, and no one treatment works for everyone. You may need to try various treatments or combinations of treatments before you find an approach that relieves your symptoms.

I hope this book has been a useful guide to you in helping you deal with your IC symptoms and hopefully help put you on the road to recovery and a worry free, pain free life. I feel even if you got one thing out of this book that helps you or gives you some relief it's served its purpose.

If you think it can help others, you can leave a review here:

https://www.amazon.com/dp/B01CFTDX4I

STICK TO IT AND GIVE IT TIME!!!

I wish you all the best in your journey; if you think this book has helped you and may help others in your shoes please leave a review.

Lightning Source UK Ltd.
Milton Keynes UK
UKHW022203040119
335040UK00025B/1367/P